The Patient's Guide

Biopsy

Adam E. M. Eltorai, MD, PhD
Omowunmi Ajibola, MD
Terrance T. Healey, MD

Praeclarus Press, LLC

www.PraeclarusPress.com

Praeclarus Press, LLC
2504 Sweetgum Lane
Amarillo, Texas 79124 USA
806-367-9950
www.PraeclarusPress.com

DISCLAIMER
The information contained in this publication is advisory only and is not intended to replace sound clinical judgment or individualized patient care. The author disclaims all warranties, whether expressed or implied, including any warranty as the quality, accuracy, safety, or suitability of this information for any particular purpose.

ISBN: 978-1-946665-31-7
©2019 Omowunmi Ajibola. All rights reserved.
Email: omowunmiajibola@gmail.com

Cover Design: Ken Tackett
Developmental Editing: Kathleen Kendall-Tackett
Copy Editing: Chris Tackett
Layout & Design: Nelly Murariu

CONTENTS

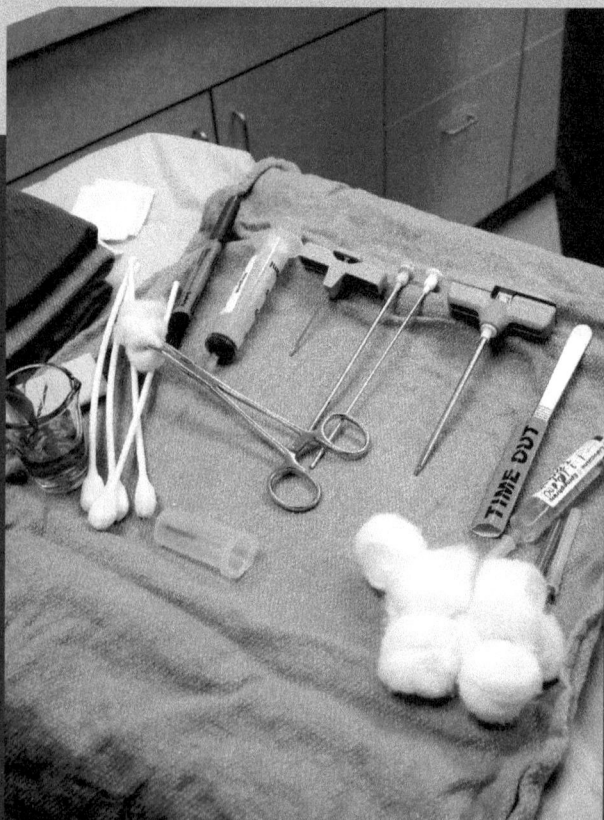

WHAT IS A BIOPSY?

A biopsy is a minimally invasive procedure in which a piece of tissue from any part of your body is obtained and sent for testing.

This is usually done with image-guided assistance, such as with an ultrasound or CT scan. They are usually performed by interventional radiologists.

Why is a biopsy performed?

There are many reasons why a biopsy is performed. If you are found to have a mass in your body and the doctors are unsure of what it is, and prior imaging studies or bloodwork haven't been able to narrow things down, they will want a biopsy to sample the mass and send it for testing to figure out what it is. It is used to determine whether said mass is benign, malignant, or cancerous.

Further testing, such as genetic testing or immune testing, is also done on the tissue samples obtained. It is usually used as a first diagnostic step. Almost any organ can be biopsied. It can also be used to evaluate for metastatic disease in cases where the initial cancer has spread. It is also used to diagnose other conditions, such as infection, inflammatory diseases, or autoimmune disease.

HOW DO I PREPARE FOR THE PROCEDURE?

M ost biopsies are done in an outpatient setting. Preparation for the procedure begins from talking to the doctor performing the procedure. The doctor should explain to you what the procedure is, as well as the risks and benefits of doing the procedure.

You should let the doctor know what medications you are taking, as the doctor needs to know which medications can be taken and which ones need to be stopped before the procedure, and if they do need to be stopped, how before the procedure to stop the medications.

It is also important to discuss how soon after the procedure when the medications can be restarted. Medications such as blood thinners are important to know.

Depending on where the mass being biopsied is, you may get some sedation. If so, then you will be advised not to have any food after midnight.

Take a bath or shower before the procedure.

Avoid using scented lotion or perfumes.

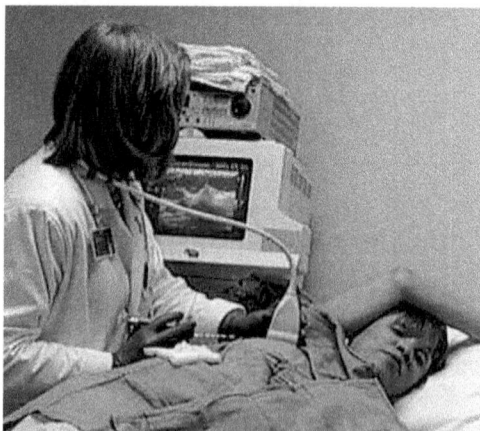

WHAT KIND OF EQUIPMENT IS USED?

There is different equipment needed, depending on what is being biopsied. In general, a long, hollow needle is used to obtain the tissue sample. It can be attached to a syringe, a barrel, or other container that holds the tissue sample. Other equipment to help with obtaining the tissue sample includes access needles and vacuum-assisted devices. Depending on the imaging modality used, any one of the following machines may be present: ultrasound machine, fluoroscopy machine, CT scanner, or MRI machine. Other equipment includes a radiographic table and a monitor to help see the images, and equipment to help monitor vital signs, such as pulse oximetry and blood pressure machines, as well as IV medications that will be administered. Other staff will be present, such as nurses, CT technicians, and anesthesiologists.

WHAT IS THE BIOPSY PROCEDURE PROCESS?

As mentioned above, the procedure is usually performed by an interventional radiologist. Before the procedure is done, the doctor will have reviewed the images and determined the best way to access the mass/area to be biopsied without hitting any major organs or vessels. Depending on that, you will either lay prone (on your stomach or supine, or on your back) on the radiographic table. A nurse will insert an IV line into a vein in your hand or arm; this will be used to administer medication and fluids. If sedation is needed, sedation medication is given through the IV. You will be connected to monitors

A local anesthetic is given superficially and into the deep tissues.

to monitor your blood pressure, oxygen level, and heart rate. The area where the procedure is to be done is cleaned and made sterile with a cleaning solution. Any hair overlying the area is shaved, and the area is draped with surgical drapes.

A local anesthetic is given superficially and into the deep tissues. Using image guidance, the needle is directed to the area of biopsy. Multiple tissue samples are obtained. Sometimes, there may be a technician from the pathology lab who looks at the tissue samples to ensure that they have enough samples and to make sure the samples are of good quality.

After the samples are taken, the needle is removed, and pressure is held on the skin to prevent bleeding, after which a dry sterile dressing is put on.

WHAT DOES A BIOPSY FEEL LIKE?

During the procedure, you should feel no pain due to the local anesthesia and general sedation, if it is given. You will be in deep sleep if general sedation is given. If you should feel anything during the procedure, it will be pressure. If you indicate that you are feeling any pain, more local anesthesia is given. If you are also receiving sedation, more sedation can also be given. The local anesthetic given lasts about 4-6 hours, so it will still be in effect when you are sent home.

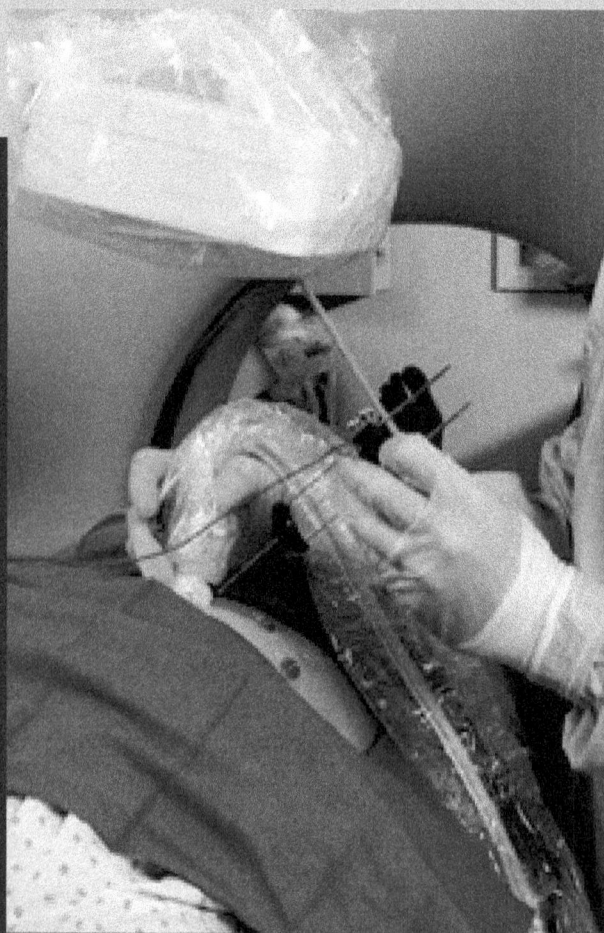

WHAT HAPPENS AFTER THE PROCEDURE?

After the procedure, you will be moved to the recovery unit and monitored for a period of time, depending on the preferences of the doctor performing the procedure. This is to make sure you tolerated the procedure well and have no acute symptoms, such as shortness of breath, hematoma, or pain at or around the area of the biopsy. During this time, the interventional radiologist will have a discussion with you and your family/loved ones as to how the procedure went. Follow-up imaging may be done to make sure no acute complications have occurred. Afterward, you will be sent home, usually the same day. Usually, no restrictions are placed on you afterwards. You can resume your daily activities as you see fit.

How do I know the results of the biopsy?

The tissue samples obtained are sent to the lab for further testing. That lab may be in house, or it may be another facility. Thus, the results from the tests performed on the tissue samples obtained may take a couple of days to come back. Your doctor will give you a call when your results are out. You should have a discussion with your doctor to go over the results and make sure you understand the results of the test.

WHAT ARE THE BENEFITS OF A BIOPSY?

- ✔ It is a minimally invasive way of diagnosing a disease, whether it be infection, malignancy, or an auto-immune disorder. No big incision or major surgery is needed to get a tissue sample.

- ✔ It is an outpatient procedure, so you can go home the same day the procedure is done.

- ✔ A needle biopsy is less painful than the surgical option, and also has faster recovery.

WHAT ARE THE RISKS OF A BIOPSY?

⚠ Any procedure that involves piercing the skin has a risk of infection and bleeding.

⚠ Depending on what part of the body is being biopsied, there could be accidental injury to adjacent structures. For instance, if a lung nodule is being biopsied, then there is a chance of pneumothorax. Or if the mass is in the abdomen, then there is a chance of hematoma or perforation of a bowel.

⚠ You, as the patient, should ensure that these, as well as the alternatives, are discussed with you by your doctor.

WHAT ARE THE LIMITATIONS OF A BIOPSY?

There are a few limitations. One is that sometimes, the tissue samples obtained may either not be good enough for testing, or too little of the sample may be obtained. Sometimes, the tissue sample obtained may be normal tissue and not from the area of interest. Sometimes, testing from the sample may not yield the answers wanted.

Another issue is that the mass has to be visible on imaging modalities, and it has to be a certain size to get good enough samples.

FREQUENTLY ASKED QUESTIONS

How long does it take?

It takes about 30-45 minutes. Including setting you up, it could take an hour to an hour and a half.

What happens if the tissue samples are not good enough?

This is a discussion you have to have with your doctor. You may need to undergo the procedure again to get more samples.

Can I come alone?

While you may come alone, it is recommended that someone comes with you and you have a

ride home, if you are receiving
sedation. It is also nice to
have someone with you while
going through an emotionally
stressful time.

What happens if there are complications?

If there are acute complications
that need to be dealt with, you
will need to stay a little longer.
If they become more serious,
you may be sent to the hospital
if you are at an outpatient site.

Will I be exposed to radiation?

Depending on the imaging
device used to view the
mass, you may be exposed to
radiation. If an ultrasound or
MRI machine is being used to
view the image, then there is
no radiation exposure.
If fluoroscopy or CT is used as
image guidance, there is some
radiation exposure.

GLOSSARY

INFLAMMATORY DISEASE

A disease in which the process of inflammation the body used to ward off infection or wounds ends up causing damage to normal cells.

AUTOIMMUNE DISEASE

A disease in which the body's immune system attacks the normal cells in the body.

ANESTHETICS

Medications that induce a temporary loss of consciousness or awareness.

INTERVENTIONAL RADIOLOGIST

A medical doctor who is trained in performing minimally invasive procedures using imaging techniques, such as X-rays and CTs.

PATHOLOGY TECHNICIAN

A person who is trained to assist the pathologist in the pathology lab.

PATHOLOGY LAB

Clinical laboratory where laboratory analysis of bodily fluids and tissue samples are done.

MINIMALLY INVASIVE

Procedure that is done through a small incision in the skin.

ANESTHESIOLOGIST

A type of doctor who specializes in giving anesthesia medicine.

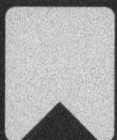

ADDITIONAL RESOURCES

Radiologyinfo.org
http://Radiologyinfo.org

Patient.info
http://Patient.info

Mayoclinic.org
Mayoclinic.org/patient-care-and-health-information

MY CONTACTS

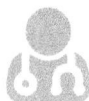

NAME

CONTACT

NAME

CONTACT

NAME

CONTACT

NAME

CONTACT

MY APPOINTMENTS

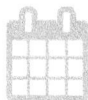

MONDAY
Date:
_____

THURSDAY
Date:
_____

TUESDAY
Date:
_____

FRIDAY
Date:
_____

WEDNESDAY
Date:
_____

SATURDAY
Date:
_____

MY QUESTIONS

MY QUESTIONS

MY QUESTIONS

MY QUESTIONS

MY QUESTIONS

MY NOTES

MY NOTES

MY NOTES

MY NOTES

MY NOTES